CPAP

Sidekick

CPAP made simple

By: RT4ME

Dedication

This book is for all of you out there, who just want sincere, honest advice. No bias, no secret motives…please enjoy.

Table of Contents

RT = Latin for Respiritus Therapitus . . . we made this

up.

An RT is a respiratory therapist!

Breathing is our business.

Chapter 1

Why did we write this book?

Greetings from RT4ME! We treat and assist patients who have different kinds of sleep apnea. The most common treatment is continuous positive airway pressure, otherwise known as CPAP. Nowadays, almost everyone knows somebody who uses CPAP, or "CPACK" or "sleep apnea machines," or simply put, "that machine." But very few people know what it all means, what to expect, how to troubleshoot problems, and the who, what, when, where, why, and hows of life with CPAP.

We help patients every day who don't know the basics, even though they own machines and are putting their faith in them. The main reason? They haven't been told the proper information by their health team. This has led us to ask several questions: Why is this information being kept from people? Why isn't there a clear and concise guide that sums up everything that a regular person needs to know when they live with sleep apnea and/or a CPAP machine? Why do patients need to ask their medical suppliers for information about when to buy new equipment and how to use it, when the information could be biased? If someone is telling me to buy things ASAP, but I am buying the things from them, is that good advice for both of us?

We at RT4ME have seen every mask, machine, tube, and circumstance that you could think of! We think that as a CPAP patient yourself, or as a person who cares about one, you deserve to know the right information, in the right way, when you want to know it. To sum it up, the *CPAP Sidekick* is CPAP MADE SIMPLE. Give it a read, trust in the words and practices described within, and take the stress out of understanding your CPAP machine. Getting the right information shouldn't break the bank!

Trust us, we're not doctors!

The RTs at RT4ME☺

Chapter 2

Sleep apnea? What's that?

Well, you've gone and done it now . . . you finally went to the sleep lab because you snore, or have morning headaches, or stop breathing at night, or because your wife/husband has kicked you out of bed . . . and now you have sleep apnea. But what does that mean?

Well, there are two kinds of sleep apnea: central and obstructive. Central sleep apnea is rare—it's when your brain decides to go on a minivacation and doesn't tell your body to breathe. Obstructive is the most common form of sleep apnea—it's when during your most important periods of deep sleep your throat relaxes and closes on itself. It's gravity letting us down! Every time this happens, air cannot get to your lungs and you lose oxygen.

Think of your airway as a highway from outside your body to your lungs, and every time your throat closes, it won't allow traffic through *or* it's down to one pitiful lane and barely anything gets through. Everyone has experienced this on the highway, and we all know how useless and frustrating it is! Imagine how your body feels after years and years of poor oxygen traffic.

So, when your throat closes up, it's called an "event," which sounds superfancy, but in reality, this is an event that you don't want to attend. The number of events that you have per hour is called the AHI (also known as the Apnea-Hypopnea Index). The medical community likes to have acronyms for everything, so believe us when we say we feel your pain.

Let's make CPAP simple: apnea = total blockage of the highway and hypopnea = down to one lane of the highway. The number of events that you have per hour, or your AHI, determines if you have obstructive sleep apnea (OSA) and/or how "bad" it is.

AHI (Apnea-Hypopnea Index)

<5 = no sleep

apnea 5–15 = mild

15–30 = moderate

>30 = severe

Can you imagine your throat closing thirty times an hour for your entire sleep cycle!? We sure can, because we see it every day. Yes, it's terrifying, and yes, it needs treatment. But

do not fear, you're not going to drop tomorrow, and this certainly is not a death sentence. It's simply a problem that needs a solution. People encounter things like this all the time, and we can adapt. A lot of our patients are petrified once they get a diagnosis of sleep apnea. They feel very isolated, and they feel skeptical too! Trust us, we have talked to our fair share of skeptics. Don't worry, everything is going to be fine, we swear on our stethoscopes!

Sleep apnea events are what make you feel so darn tired too. When your body is in its deepest and most regenerative phase of sleep is when it recharges its batteries, rests, and builds up its stores for the oncoming day. Unfortunately, this is also when your airways collapse the most often, so the body rouses from this stage and moves into a less restful stage to reopen your airways. People with sleep apnea can be "asleep" for hours at night but don't feel rested at all because they are staying out of their most restful periods of deep sleep every night. We have had so many patients come to us and say, "I could sleep for twelve hours and not feel as if I rested at all!" Now, if that kind of a night doesn't sound attractive to you, can you imagine *years* of sleeping like this?

Having years of poor sleep, as well as poor oxygenation, can really take its toll on one's body. It can lead to atrial fibrillation, irregular heart rates, heart attack, stroke, and high blood pressure, just to name a few issues that should make *anyone* with sleep apnea want to treat it. To make it simple: your body loves oxygen, so make sure it gets it.

Now that we have scared the dickens out of you . . .

The simple fact of the matter is that OSA is a real thing, it is very common, and you are not alone. The best part is that it can be treated without having to spend a lot of money, without having to put drugs into your body, and without surgery. CPAP is the most common treatment for OSA—you probably know this already, or else you wouldn't have picked up this book. We are really happy that you decided to learn about sleep apnea, and we think that by learning the basics, you will be a lot more comfortable with CPAP, its use, and your outlook on your health and wellness.

Like we said, there are many treatments for OSA, but the most common is a CPAP machine. Your doctor will give you a prescription for a certain pressure and send you on your merry way to go a buy a machine and mask. Do you want to know what this "thing" will do for you? Read on dear friend, read on!

Chapter 3

What is a CPAP machine?

CPAP stands for "continuous positive airway pressure," but do us a favour and just call it CPAP. A CPAP machine keeps your throat open during sleep by providing a flow of air pressure. The machine doesn't breathe for you—you can't give up completely, you have to still do *some* of the work. Think of the machine as a doorstop that holds your throat open, allowing you to breathe smoothly and uninterruptedly. The air pressure is measured in centimetres of water (cm H_2O), and this is why your prescription will say "9 cm H_2O" or "5 cm," etc. Why is this? Because ventilators that are used in hospitals by RTs like us are measured in cm H_2O! And gosh, we sure do hate change. Just go with it.

And remember, folks, a pressure of 5 cm H_2O has nothing to do with how much water you put in your humidifier or how high to set the humidifier! If this means nothing to you, please keep reading, as it will all be as clear as mud eventually. And if you are simply skimming this, stop it!

But my friend has something called an APAP, or an auto machine. Is that CPAP?

Yes! And no. Sometimes people use a machine called an APAP, or an automatic positive airway pressure machine. What's the difference? Well, CPAP is only one pressure all the time, for example, 10 cm H_2O. That is the only pressure that the machine goes to during your entire night of sleep; it does not change. An APAP machine sets two bookends of pressure, let's say 5–15 cm H_2O, and the machine will move between those two bookends throughout the night, depending on what your body is asking for. Some people need a different pressure depending on where in their sleep cycle they are, or if they sleep on their back vs. on their side, so an APAP can adapt to that. How, you ask?

MAGIC.

APAP users, CPAP users, and anyone who is using a

machine like these can benefit from the advice we give in this

book. So, if you are an APAP user, or even a Bilevel user, when

we write CPAP we mean all y'all.

What are the parts of the machine?

Think of your CPAP machine as a glorified leaf blower,

but this leaf blower has two halves: a motor and a humidifier.

The motor portion sucks in room air and directs it to you (and

your airway) at your prescribed pressure. The air that travels

from the motor can be as dry as a chip, and this is why your

CPAP is equipped with a humidifier. Inside of the humidifier is

a water tub that needs refilling every day. You can adjust your

humidity as you see fit based on your comfort . . . and don't

worry there is no wrong answer—if there was a wrong answer,

then you wouldn't be allowed to touch the humidifier setting!

Your tube (or hose) will then connect from the humidifier to your mask. The tube is roughly two metres (six feet) long, and will attach from any machine to any mask. There are standard tubes and heated tubes, and typically, CPAP machines come with standard tubes. Heated tubes are usually an upgrade, and are a bit more expensive, but will give you better humidity and a cleaner tube long term. Not every heated tube will work with every machine though, so if you are going to invest in one, get some advice from your CPAP provider or the manufacturer first.

The tube attaches to your mask, and we are going to talk in another chapter about masks and how you will feel while using your CPAP.

Most machines nowadays have a cellular modem inside them, which allows your doctor or provider to monitor you remotely, and if needed, they can troubleshoot if you have any issues, and can alter your pressure if a change is ordered. The modem should not cost you a thing, so watch out for cash grabs, because the modem is built into the machine by the manufacturer. The modem provides a great connection between you and your provider, and will save you the time and energy of dragging yourself out of the house to have your pressure adjusted or to have a usage download done for your physician.

Also built into the machine is an SD card for tracking data, and a filter that sits inside the air intake of the machine. Like any ventilation system, similar to the HVAC you have in your home, your CPAP machine has its own filter that is unique to it.

These are the basic parts of the machine. You should be shown all of these at the time of setup, and if you were not shown these basics, then you may want to call your provider for a re-education session or think of finding an alternative to your current provider as this information should be made available to you at the time of purchase. Luckily, there are hundreds of CPAP providers all over North America, so if one isn't meeting your needs, then you can shop around.

Chapter 4

What will CPAP feel like?

CPAP will feel like nothing you have ever experienced before. CPAP isn't uncomfortable, it's just new, and new situations simply require that people adapt. It will take some time; most people need a week or two to get used to it. If it takes you a week, or if it takes you a month, it is *your* journey and everybody has their own unique journey. Here are some tips and pointers for you to read when things get tough. Stick with it because you can do it!

The first thing that you want to do when you get your mask on and your machine is running is to get the rhythm of your breathing. Your machine usually won't go to your full pressure right at the beginning; it will start at a lower pressure. This is called "ramp." Older machines used to go straight to the full therapy pressure, but a lot of people found that trying to fall asleep on full pressure was difficult. When "ramp" is turned on your machine, you begin at a lower pressure than your prescription pressure, and over time the machine slowly ramps up to your full pressure. This should make it easier for you to fall asleep.

As you practice your breathing and get your rhythm, you will notice that breathing out against the "leaf blower" is a unique and strange feeling. You will get used to this, and all machines have the ability to back off on the pressure when you breathe out. Each manufacturer has its own name for its pressure relief feature. Ask your provider if your pressure relief is turned on, as this will help with your comfort.

Another key point to remember is that air is very lazy—it isn't going to do any work in your airway if it enters your nose and then you open your mouth. Lazy air is going to take the first corner and rush out of your mouth instead of helping you out. This is why you need to practice breathing *only* through your nose. This will take time. We encourage people to practice using their CPAP while they are watching television or reading. Practice makes perfect!

One of the most common questions that we get is, "Do I have to wear it for eight hours at night?" Who actually sleeps eight hours per night? We don't know anybody. We think that people who sleep eight hours a night are like unicorns—they don't exist. But seriously, we advise trying to get four hours of CPAP use (or more) each and every night. Your doctor has prescribed you this therapy for a very good reason, so you really need to use it. If you can use the machine for four good hours, you can get a lot of the benefits of CPAP and get enough data to know how effective CPAP has been for you. You will be amazed at the information these machines can give us!

If you talk while using your CPAP, you will instantly turn

into Darth Vader. This is okay; don't be afraid, just use the Force. You may feel some discomfort at the beginning if you try to talk while wearing your CPAP, but you will get used to it. If you try to breathe through your mouth while wearing your CPAP nasal mask or pillow, it will feel as though you have something caught in your throat or are choking, so you need to practice using your nose for breathing in and out, and not your mouth.

Think of it like a traffic intersection in the city. Imagine lots of cars waiting to go, and then suddenly all of the lights go green, in every direction. You are going to have a serious problem—the cars are going to run into each other and create big collisions.

Well, this is what happens when you have CPAP sending air through your nose but you also give the green light to your mouth! We like to think that this is the only time in life that you are allowed to tell someone to "shut your mouth."

The CPAP tube is roughly two metres (six feet) long, and a lot of masks add extra tube so you have lots of leeway if you need to roll back and forth while you sleep. Keep the machine level with you on the bed or lower; don't keep it up high above you! If water collects in the tube you want gravity to bring it back down to the machine, and not down to your face!

The number one piece of feedback that we can give you is to relax. You are in control, you set the pace, and if you are ever feeling overwhelmed you can *always* take the mask off. Using the CPAP machine will take time and practice, but you can do it. We believe in you. If you need coaching, get in touch with your doctor or health team. Everyone wants you to be comfortable and relaxed.

Chapter 5

25

Masks

Masks . . . which one is the best one?

Well, who is the greatest artist? Who is the best actress? What is the best running shoe?

The answers to *all* of the above questions are very subjective, and to answer them simply: to each his own. Every individual person has a different face, and therefore a different experience with the various masks that are on the market. We can't tell you which is the best mask, but what we sure can tell you is that the mask is the deal breaker for your CPAP therapy. If you don't like the mask, you ain't gonna wear it! So let's start with some basics.

The three most common styles of masks are:

1) Full face mask (covers your nose and mouth)

2) Nasal mask (covers your nose)

3) Nasal pillow mask (rests in your nostrils)

Let's begin with the biggest fear that people have—full face masks (FFMs).

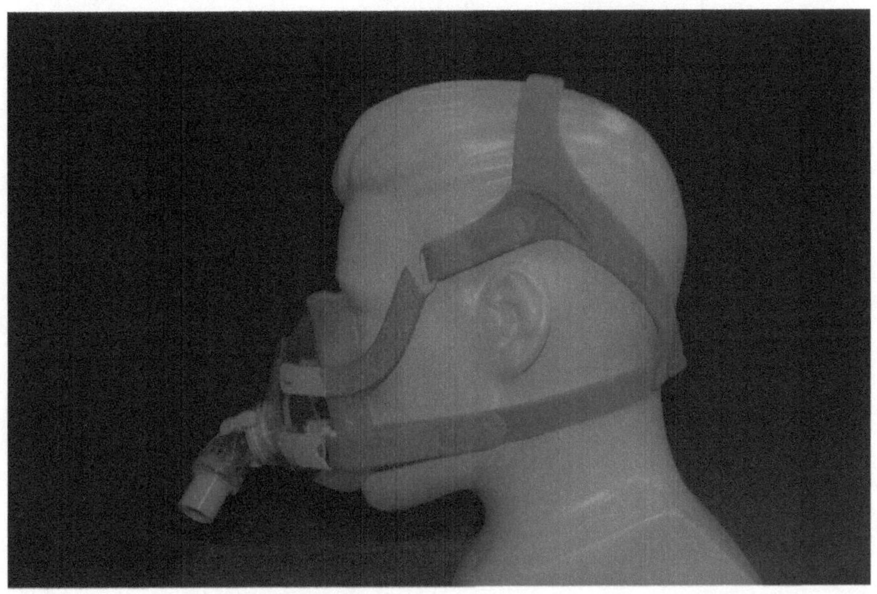

Full Face Mask

Key points:

- Covers your nose and mouth.

- Is heavier, more expensive, and more substantial than nasal masks and nasal pillow masks.

- Can be challenging to create a good seal on the face; leaks are common.

- Difficult to speak while using.

- Can sometimes cause nose bridge breakdown/redness on the nose.

- Designed for patients who continue to mouth breathe even after starting CPAP therapy.

EXTRA CREDIT

"Well, I'm a mouth breather, so I need the full face mask."

False. Luckily, this is more fiction than fact! The biggest misconception with masks is that you need a full face mask if you are a mouth breather. The majority of people with sleep apnea sleep with their mouths open *because they have sleep apnea.*

Why? Because we are clever animals, and animals adapt. We learned to open our mouth when our airway closes because by doing this, our throat opens up! So, once we start CPAP therapy and use simple nasal or nasal pillow masks, after two weeks or so, we don't open our mouth while we sleep anymore because the CPAP is keeping our airway open! It's a CPAP miracle!

Now, back to where we left off . . .

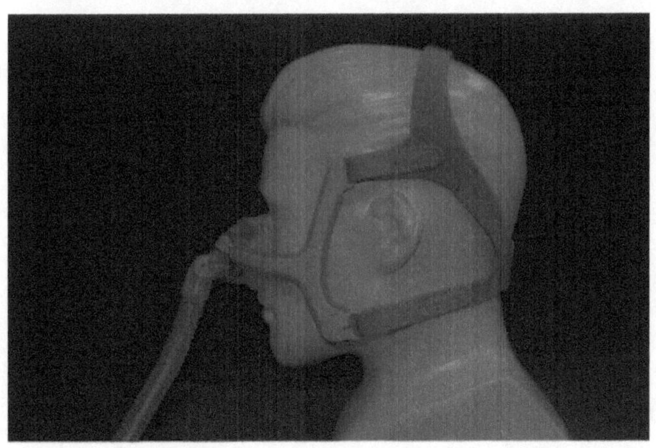

Nasal Mask

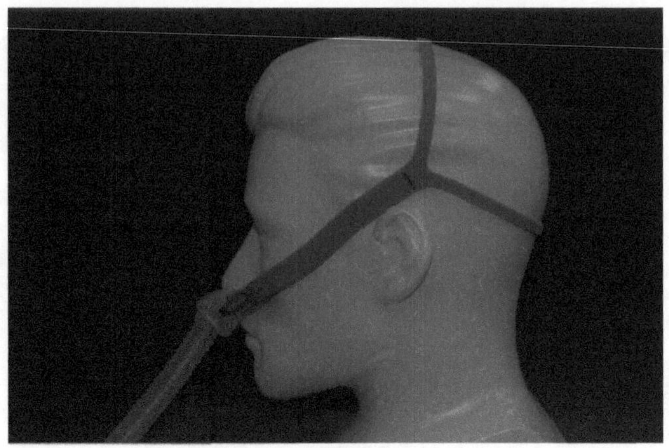

Nasal Pillow Mask

Key points:

- The most common masks on the market today.

- They are lightweight, easy to use, and more affordable than full face masks.

- Very few leaks.

- Can speak and drink while using these masks.

- Can sometimes create nose bridge breakdown/redness.

Whatever mask you end up using, it needs to be comfortable and easy for you to use. CPAP users happily strap one of these on every night and never have a problem. There are many models to choose from, so it's nice to have a health team available to help you pick the one that's right for you. Most RTs can look at your face and nose and give you great advice about what mask you should try. The other beauty is that most companies that sell masks have a one-time exchange policy (within thirty days), so if you dislike the mask you went home with the first time, you can swap it for another one, no quibbles! Most people, once they find a mask that they love, stick with it. Like we said, the mask is the deal breaker for using the machine; if you don't like the mask, it won't matter if you can tolerate the machine pressure because you won't want that thing on your face!

Some of the key things to remember:

1) If you have any issues with anxiety or claustrophobia, it might be good to try some nasal pillow masks. Sometimes the nasal masks and full face masks can be overwhelming because the headgear is more substantial and heavier. And that's okay! Some people are scared of clowns, some people aren't, so there is no wrong way to feel about your mask.

2) As the type of mask grows in size, the greater the chance of leak. What is this leak we speak of? Well, "leak" is when the mask isn't sealing well to your face and air escapes out the sides. This can be really annoying—it can blow into your eyes or even make embarrassing noises! And remember, we got into this

CPAP thing to *stop* making noise while we sleep. If the leak is large enough, it can also render the therapy useless—if the air isn't going into your throat because it's leaking out of the sides of the mask, then what's the point? So, fit is extremely important, which leads us to the third point.

3) If you have to tighten your mask so much that its straps leave you looking like a raccoon, it is not the right mask for you. You should not feel any pain, you shouldn't have lines on your face, and you shouldn't have any skin breakdown on the bridge of your nose. We always say that it's a fine balance between tight enough to seal and loose enough that you don't go to work in the morning and everyone says, "Hey, Charlie, how's that new CPAP mask?" If you find

that your mask is leaving marks on your face or neck, there are gel pads for the bridge of your nose and padding for the straps; simply put, there is an accessory for everything!

4) Certain brands fit a certain way. Just like running shoe companies use the same last (or mould) for creating the fit of their shoes, CPAP mask companies have a similar fit to all of their masks. This creates brand loyalty for a lot of users, and also creates trends in terms of nose shapes and face shapes working better with certain brands. This is a great time to talk to an RT or sleep professional to get some advice or insight into choosing the right mask.

Just keep in mind, it is a free market and most likely the people

who are going to be directing you toward these expensive items

will also stand to profit from your purchase. If you are worried,

find an unbiased source of information where you can get great

advice on all things CPAP.

Chapter 6

What are these things called!?

One of the biggest challenges that our patients face is learning the *names* of everything! When they call or email us, they will call pieces of their equipment all sorts of different things! "The hook thing on the front of the face part," or "You know that part on the face?" and "The piece of fabric."

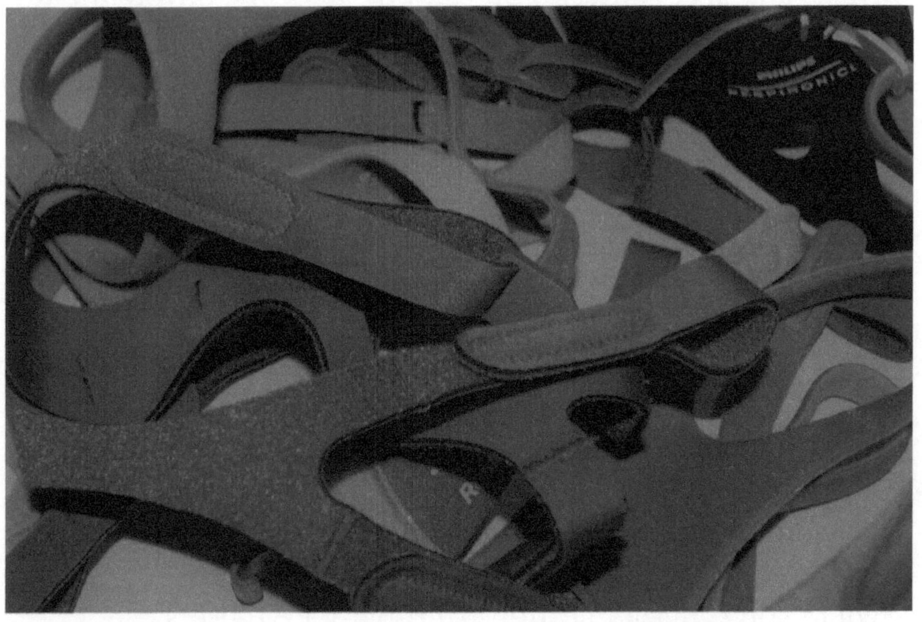

Does this picture sum up your knowledge of CPAP parts?

Well, dear CPAP user, our pledge of "CPAP MADE SIMPLE" is at its most applicable in this chapter! We are going to go over everything that you need to know—name names *and* provide you with photos so you will become fluent in CPAP! You're welcome.

Do you know what else is superawesome about CPAP masks and accessories? You can buy all of the different parts separately, so if you want to save some money, or if you snap one of the small pieces in the middle of the night, fear not, you can order each of these things on their own.

Read this chapter to learn all of the lingo, and if you still aren't sure about what to order, or how to order it, ask your provider or hop online—there are plenty of CPAP forums where you can ask questions of other CPAP users.

Now, sit back and enjoy the slideshow!

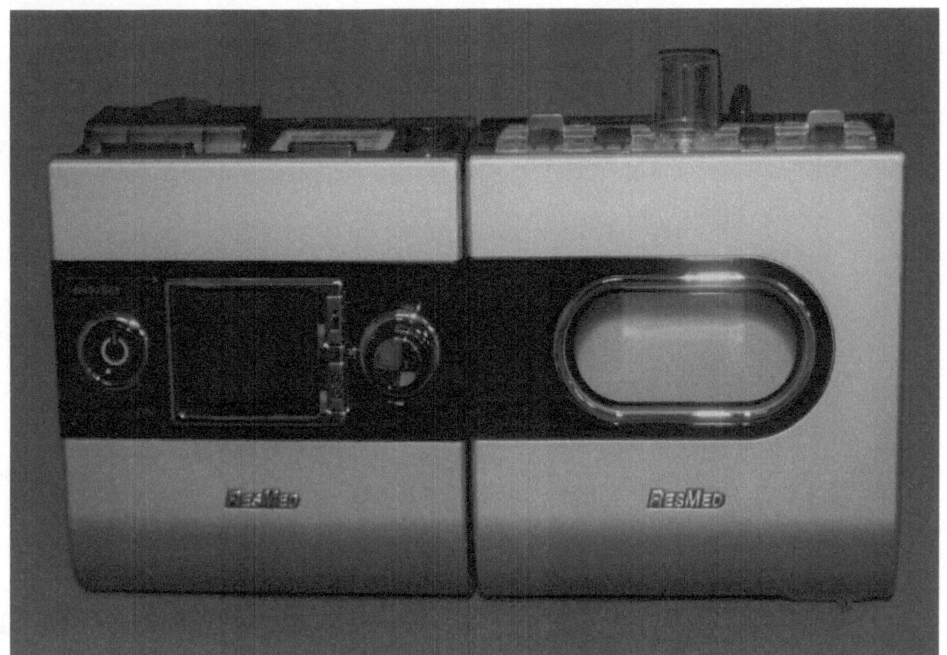

ResMed S9 Elite or AutoSet

Key points:

- Usually have a motor side and a humidifier side (like the above photo).

- The motor side sucks in the air through the air intake and then shoots it back out at the prescription pressure.

- The air then travels through the humidifier and becomes humidified.

- The tube connects to the humidifier and then travels to the mask.

- Some models are one solid unit.

- Machines usually come with a three-year warranty.

- Some newer models are equipped with a cellular modem so that your provider can download your usage data and monitor your progress. Machines will come with an SD card, air filter, tube, and water tub at time of purchase.

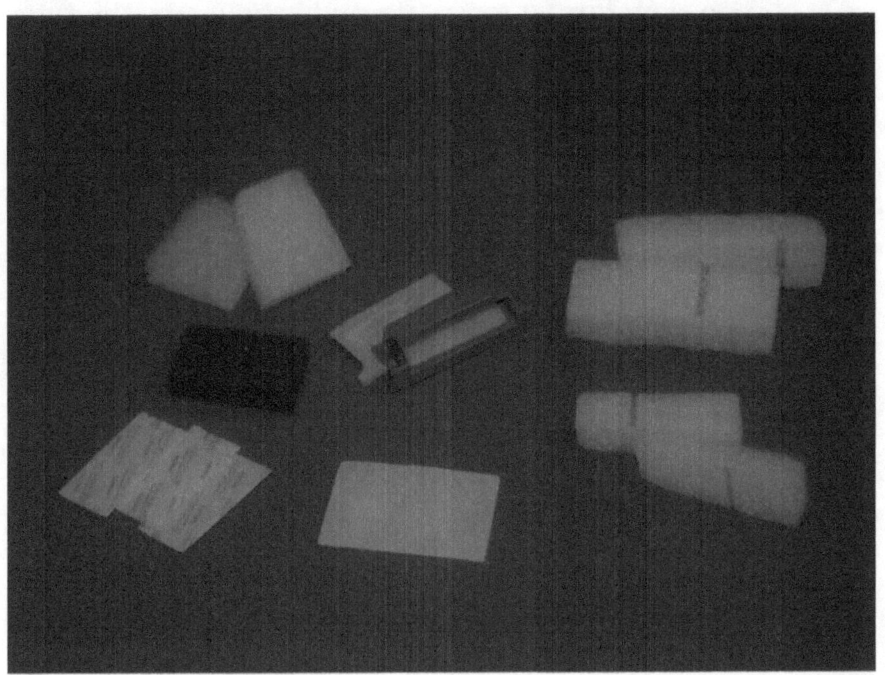

Key points:

- This is the first line of defence for cleanliness as this filters out particles in the air before you breathe them in.

- Located at the back or side of the machine at the air intake.

- Needs to be replaced every 3–6 months, depending on how dirty it gets—if you live in a city, the filter can get dirty faster—and best way to know is to look at it! Does it look gross? *Replace it. You are breathing through this!*

- Some models have two filters that go in at the same time—a disposable one for smaller particles and a reusable one for larger particles. Check your instruction manual or ask for help!

The air goes from the intake to the filter to the motor to the humidifier, so let's go there next!

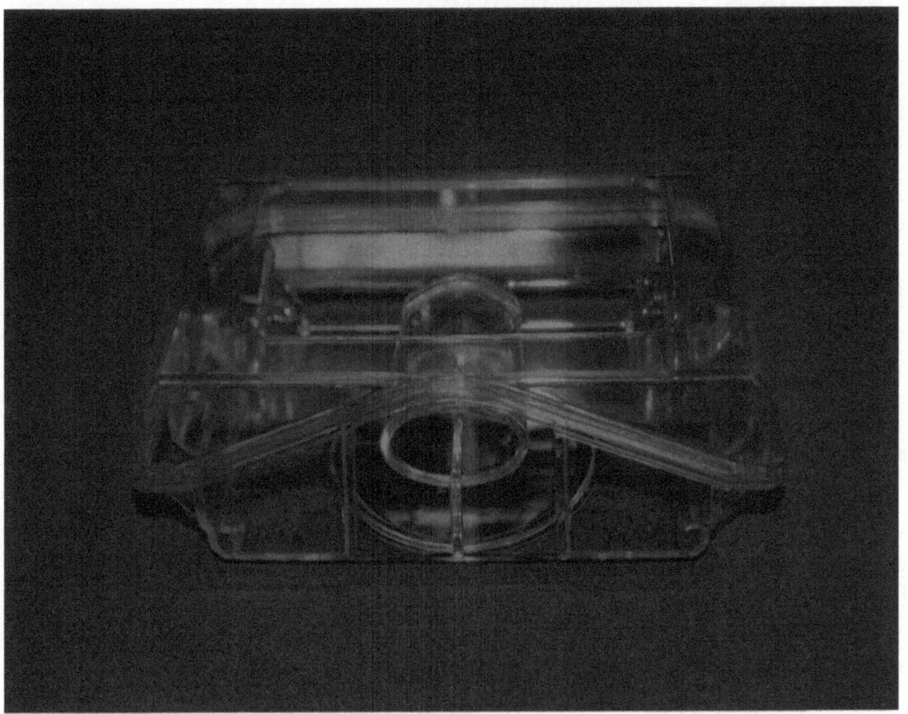

Water tub for the Philips Respironics DreamStation.

Key points:

- Every machine has a water tub.

- These are also known as the water chamber, humidifier tub, humidifier chamber, or water pot.

- Every machine has its own unique tub, so you need to order the right one.

- Usually should be filled with distilled water; some models are upgraded and can use tap water.

- Needs to be emptied every morning after use and refilled each night before use.

- Needs to be washed in warm water and mild soap or vinegar once a week.

- Replace the tub once a year if you can.

The air then travels from the water tub to the tube, so let's look at the two kinds of tubes that you can get! Onward!

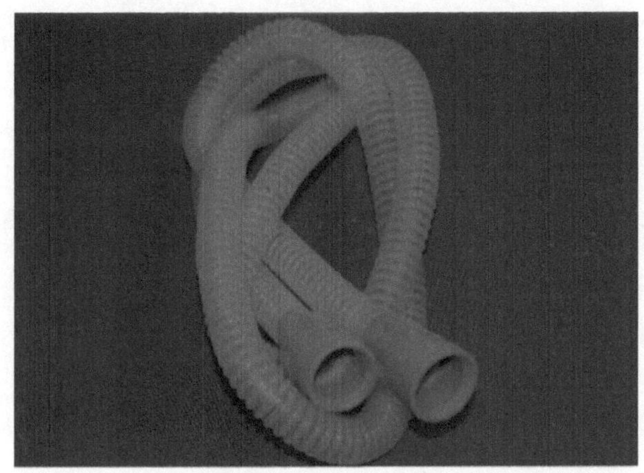

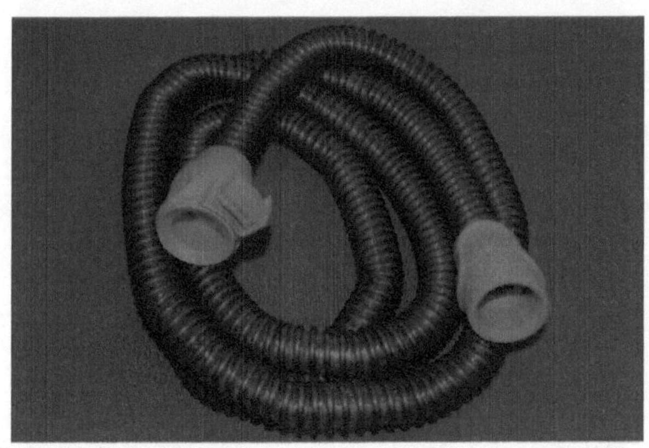

Top and Bottom: standard tube; heated tube.

Key points:

- Also called hoses, circuits, or heated hoses.

- Two kinds: standard and heated.

- Standard comes with the machine, and is simply the tube that the air travels through with universal connections on the ends (22 mm); can be wide or slim in diameter.

- Heated are typically an upgraded purchase—one end will be standard so that it connects with the mask, the other end will be specific to the make and model of the CPAP machine.

- Needs to be washed in warm water and mild soap or vinegar once a week.

- Replace the tube once a year if you can.

The air travels from the tube to the mask, so let's take a look at all of the things that you need to know about the masks . . . get comfy!

There are many parts and pieces to CPAP masks, so we are going to break it down for you in simple terms and *big* photos.

We will go from:

Tubes

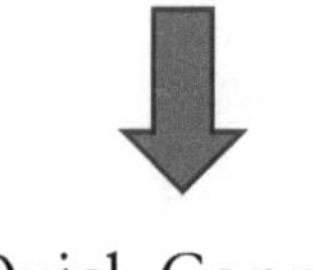

Quick Connect

Frame

Cushion

Headgear

Clip

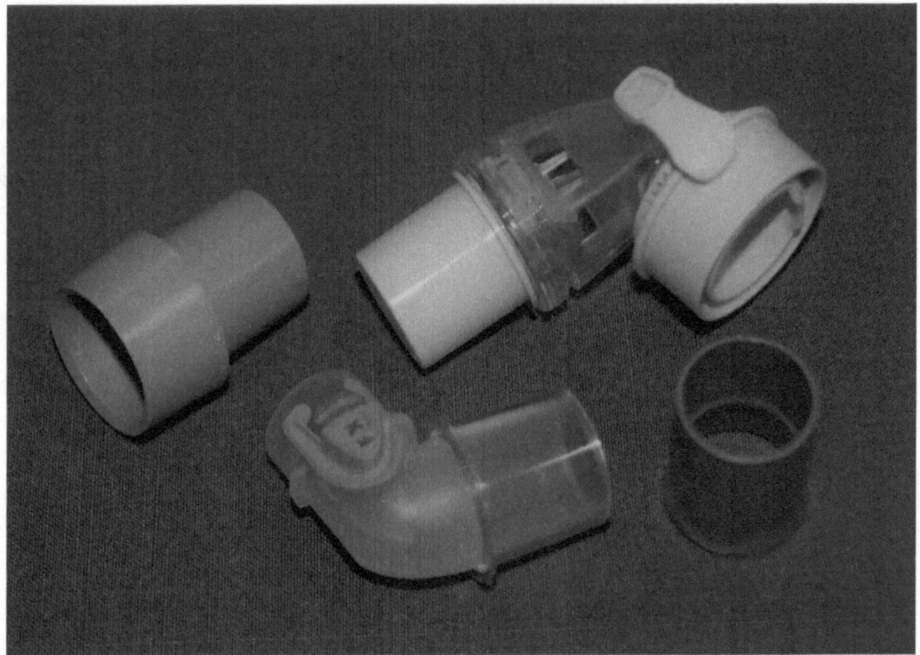

A variety of random quick connects from various masks.

Key points:

- Also called elbows, spacers, "the thing in the tube" or "the thing on the face part of the mask."

- The tube connects to this part of the mask.

- Are an easy way to detach the tube from the mask.

- Why? To go to the bathroom, to check on the kids, to get a drink of water.

- Either clips or snaps on with ease.

- Sometimes has a port for air to blow out; this is normal.

RT4ME TIP

We have seen *so many* people leave the quick connect in the end of the tube after use, and then when they buy a new tube, they toss out the quick connect with their old tube *or* they buy a new mask and the old tube won't connect because it has the old quick connect still in it! Double check this before making a trip in to see your provider!

FRAME

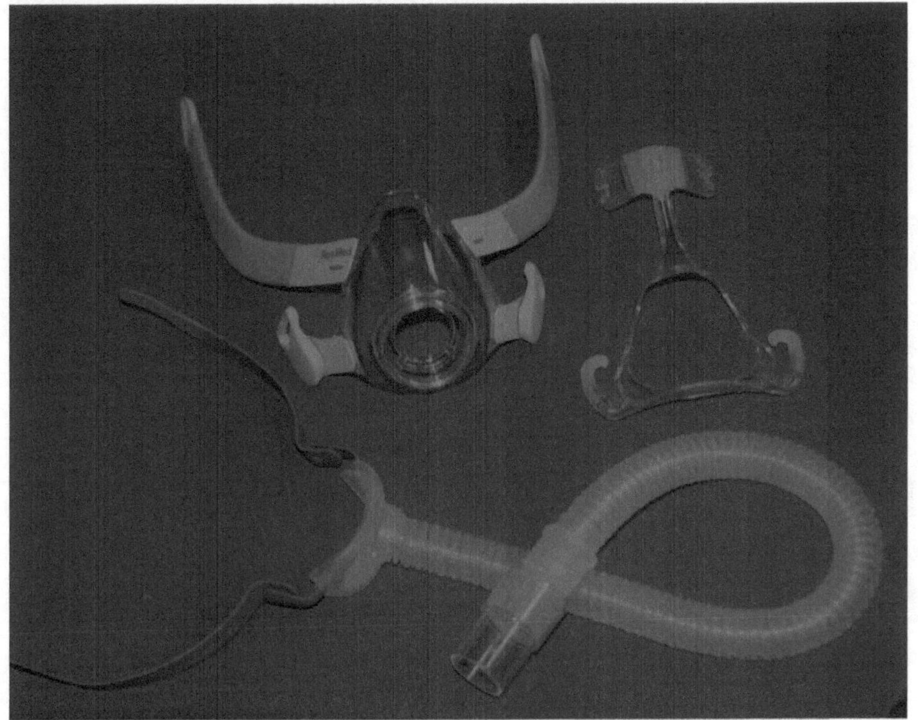

A variety of frames from different manufacturers.

Key points:

- Also called hard part, the part the tube goes on, the part where the soft thing goes, or the skeleton.

- The quick connect meets the frame, and the frame houses the cushion, which is the gel/silicone/foam part that contacts your face.

- Think of the frame as the skeleton of the mask, everything else grows from it!

- Each mask has a specific frame.

What attaches to the frame? Most importantly the *cushion*, *headgear*, and the *clips*.

Onward friend

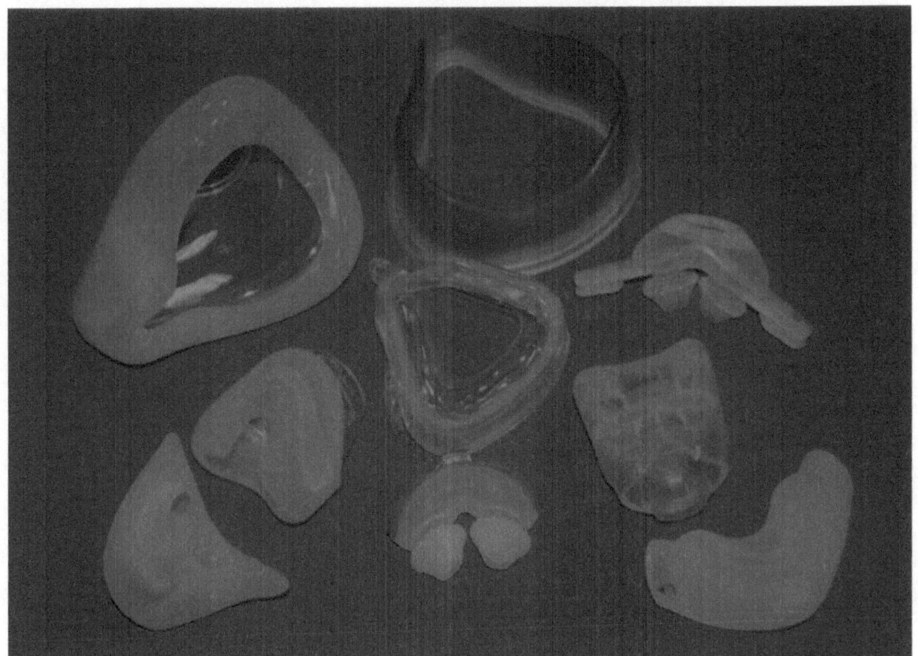

A variety of cushions from different masks.

Key points:

- Also called pillows, gel part, silicone, nosepiece, face piece, the part on your face.

- Specific to the model of mask.

- Can become brittle and/or discoloured over time due

  to skin oils.

- Can use CPAP wipes and/or alcohol-free baby wipes

  to clean each day after use.

- Attaches to the frame of the mask.

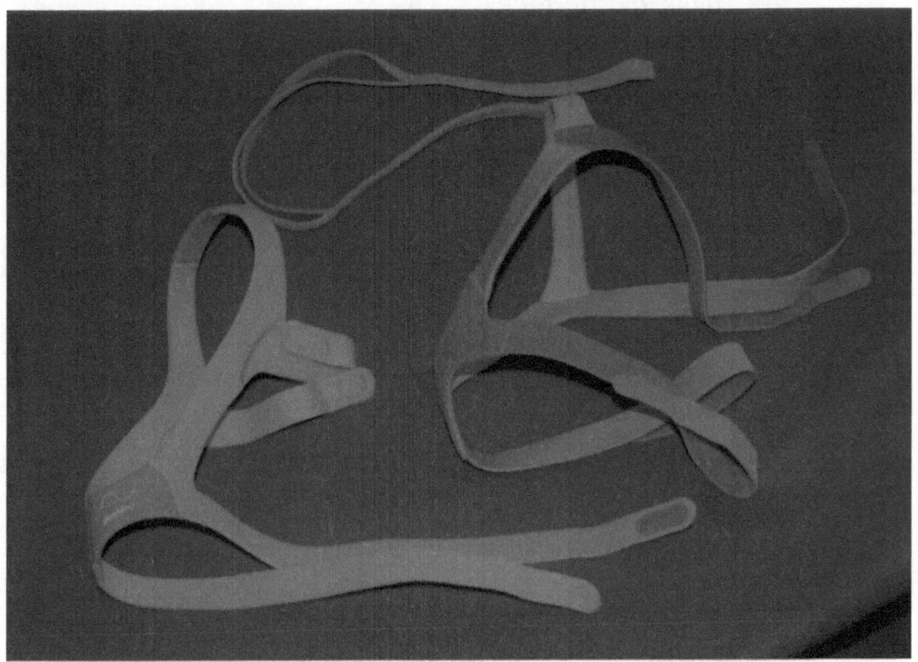

Headgear examples from three different models and styles of masks.

Key points:

- Also called straps, fabric, head part, Velcro, or material part.

- Connects to the frame via the *clips* and secures the mask to the face.

- Equipped with Velcro to tighten or loosen the headgear as needed, and it's machine washable!

Tip: Always adjust the straps in a symmetrical manner: *both* bottom straps or *both* top straps at the same time. This way, the mask is tightened or loosened evenly on the face!

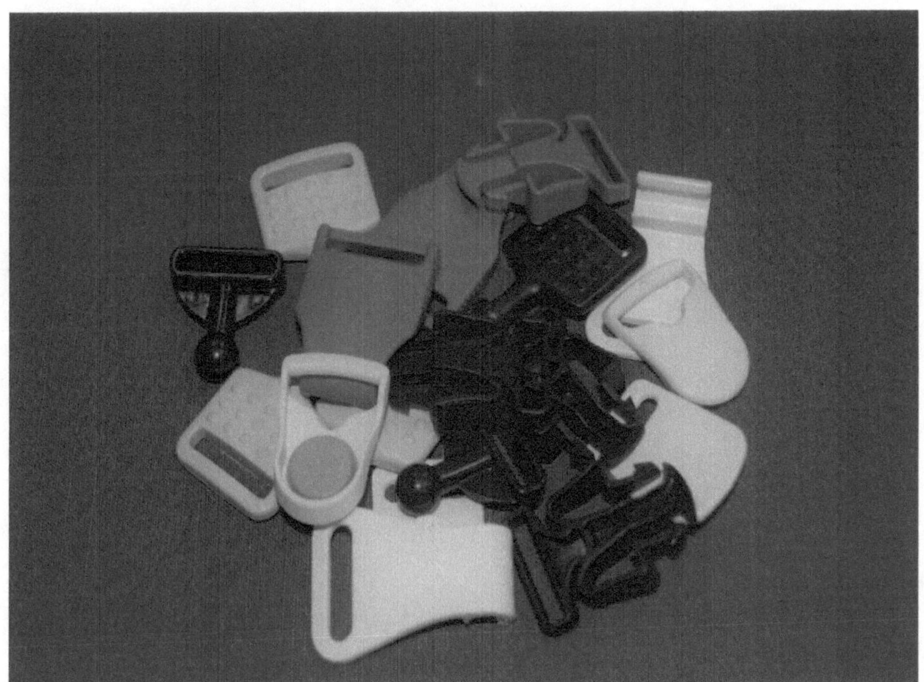

A variety of clips from many different masks and
manufacturers.

Key points:

- Also called snaps, buttons, headgear clips, joints, or

  ties.

- Specific to each mask.

- Connects the *headgear* to the *frame* with ease.

- Usually makes a "click" sound when properly attached.

- Different brands will not "play" with each other.

So, how do we know if the machine is working? If we are using it enough? If the prescribed pressure is right? Well, flip the page Curious Karen . . . we have good news for you.

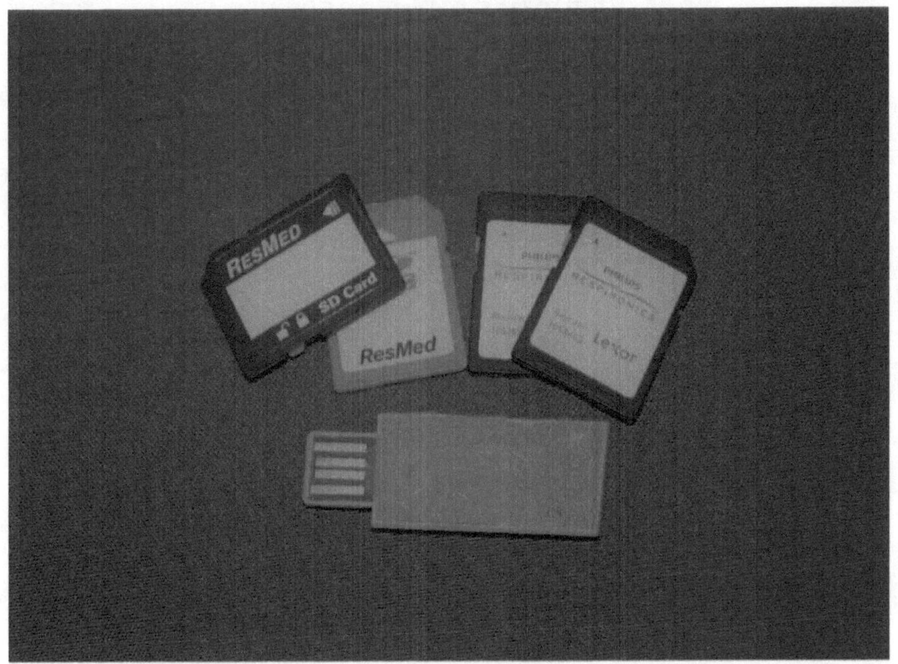

A variety of SD cards from different machines and manufacturers.

Key points:

- Also called the chip, the card, the download, the data, the microchip, or the thing in the back.

- Each machine tracks your usage and calculates useful data, which it stores on the SD card.

- Each machine has an SD card, and if you bring it to your doctor or provider, they can create a report to let you know how well the machine is working, how the mask is fitting, and even how many events per hour you are having. (This shows us that the machines are taking over the human race. Run!)

- If your provider or doctor says, "bring me a download" or "get your data" or "bring the chip," it is usually code for "have the SD card downloaded, please."

- Your provider should do this for you.

- If you damage, remove, and/or lose the card, the machine will still work just fine, so don't panic. You can buy a normal SD card from a computer store and it will work just fine.

Putting it all together!

We know, we know. That chapter was *looooong,* but at least it had photos. Each and every CPAP machine part that we outlined can be purchased separately. So, if you're on a budget, or if your dog ate your homework *and* your headgear, you can buy individual pieces of the masks.

Chapter 7

Cleaning and Maintenance

Should you clean this stuff? Your mother would have a *fit* if she heard you ask that question!

Every piece of equipment should be cleaned and replaced at certain times, and we will let you know when "best practice" says to do it . . . and by "best practice," we mean science. The reality, though, is that people forget, or they can't afford new equipment, or life just happens and then a year has gone by and they realize that their new mask is now gross. It's okay. We understand. We also understand that "CPAP Guilt" is a real thing and it's embarrassing to admit that you haven't cleaned your medical equipment.

The reality is that if you fail to keep your gear clean, lots can happen. The fit of your mask may start to become difficult because the silicone in the mask will lose its elasticity from the oils in your skin; the result is that it will start leaking. The Velcro on the headgear may start to disintegrate and then the mask will not fit correctly. The mask, tube, and water tub are an amusement park for bacteria, and could give you an infection and/or start to smell. Using nondistilled water can create a buildup of minerals on your equipment, and without regular cleaning your water tub, tube, and mask can become discoloured. Harvard University did a study that supports the practice of regularly cleaning and replacing your gear, and if Harvard says that you need to do it, you should do it.

In short, clean your stuff.

When? With what? Well, read on friend, we have got you covered…

Cleaning and Maintenance Frequency

Daily

- Change the water in your humidifier tub after *every* use—stagnant water is a playground for bacteria! Dump the water, leave the water tub empty during the day, and then refill it at night.

- If you have CPAP wipes, wipe the cushion of your mask when you wake up every day.

- CPAP wipes can be expensive, so some people save money by using alcohol-free baby wipes as a substitute, or even a cloth with warm water. The idea is to use a chemical-free source so the silicone doesn't break down . . . so go ahead, save some money!

<u>**Weekly**</u>

- Wash your mask, tube, and water tub in a sink of warm soapy water—a mild dish soap is perfect! You don't need to scrub them, just a light wash and rinse should keep your items fresh!

Tip: After rinsing out your tube, sling it over the shower curtain rod in your bathroom to drain!

<u>**Every 3–6 months**</u>

- Replace the filter in your machine. This is superimportant because the filter gets rid of all of the pollen and fluff in the air. If you have cats or smokers in the house, make it every three months or fewer. If you don't have either of these in the home, you can push it to six months!

<u>**Every year**</u>

- Replace the mask, tube, and water tub. Yes, yes, this is expensive, but guess what? These three items will still get pretty bacteria covered, even if you are doing your weekly maintenance. There are loads of online shops where you can save some money and do what's right for your health.

We know that this seems very overwhelming; sometimes our situations mean that we can't buy new stuff when it's "best practice," and all we can say is that we recommend replacing your gear, but we also recommend paying your rent and buying groceries. This is not life support, nothing is going to combust if you wait longer to get new stuff. But please, we just ask that you use your brain. Does it look or smell gross? Replace it.

Does buying supplies on the internet scare you? Do you not trust online retailers? We understand. We think that computers lie. If you need a hand ordering new gear, you can call most online shops or providers and talk to a human being, and they will help you! If your provider isn't helpful, then try another one! There are plenty of fish in the sea, and you should be able to get help from the companies that you are giving your money to . . . if not, then why are you paying them?

Chapter 8

FAQs

In this section, we have included many of the most common questions about CPAP machines that RTs get asked on a regular basis. They may be random, or they may not fit into any of the other chapters of this book. Needless to say, if we have heard a question more than five times, then the chances are that most people may wonder about these things. Without further adieu . . . enjoy!

1) *Can sleep apnea be cured or am I stuck with this machine forever?*

Well, in rare cases, obstructive sleep apnea can go away if the sufferer has OSA because of weight-related problems. More than likely, though, it is a forever diagnosis. Sleep apnea is something that you will most likely have for the rest of your life. The *good* news is that CPAP is *not* a drug, *not* painful, and *not* a treatment that changes your anatomy (i.e. surgery). There are very few "forevers" in health care that don't require drugs or surgery, so be thankful that you don't need anything invasive! You will certainly get used to the mask and machine, it will just take some time.

2) *My tube sounds like popcorn when I use it! What do I do?*

In the colder months of the year, RTs get this question the most! When your tube sounds like popcorn or like a car sputtering, there is a very simple reason: there is water trapped in your tube! How does it get there? Well, when the water in the humidifier heats up, but the tube is cold (like in the winter), condensation happens. When the air from the machine travels over these small puddles of water in the tube, it makes a weird noise. This is what you are hearing, and all you need to do is drain the water out of the tube and try to keep your tube warmer. There are a few solutions, and we will list them in ascending price:

A) Put your tube under your blankets while you sleep.

B) Lower your machine to the floor so that gravity brings the pooling water back into the humidifier.

C) Wrap the tube in a towel to keep it insulated.

D) Buy a tube wrap from your local provider, which is like a long towel with a zipper on it.

E) Buy a heated tube, which has a heated coil inside of it, from your provider.

The overall strategy, if you can see it, is to keep the temperature change from the humidifier to the tube as small as possible. Keep your tube warm and the popcorn sound will go away!

3)   *Is my CPAP safe around my pets?*

We're not going to lie, *most* pets will be fine around your
machine. The thing that you really need to keep an eye
on is your machine filter, because cat hair will clog it up
faster than any other kind of pet hair. If you don't know
where the filter is, refer back to the equipment chapter.
Also, we have frequently seen tubes that have multiple
puncture holes in them because kitties like to nibble on
them from time to time. If you have one small puncture
hole, it's probably *not* your pet, but if there are multiple
holes in a concentrated area, then Mr. Fluffers is
probably chomping on your tube when you aren't
looking!

4) *Do I need to bring this on vacation? Do I check it as luggage?*

RTs are asked this a lot when we are setting people up for the first time, whereas ongoing users rarely ask this. We usually ask our clients to get used to using the machine first, then make the decision about whether or not they want to travel with it. More often than not, people realize that they feel so much better on CPAP that they couldn't imagine not feeling rested on vacation, which is where they want to feel the most rested and rejuvenated! Always bring your CPAP with you as carry-on. Airlines *do not* count it as one of your carry-on items because it is deemed a medical device. If you check the machine with your baggage, be prepared for it to grow legs. Most airlines won't let you use the machine in the air, which some of our clients get worried about. We usually say don't fret, the seats on most airlines don't allow you to lie back far enough for your sleep apnea to occur anyway. If you are practically sitting up the whole time, you won't even need that darn thing. If lugging that bedside machine through the airport is too awkward for you, think about investing in a travel CPAP. Just google it. There are tons of models out there, and most are very lightweight, comfortable, and quiet. Most machines sold from 2008 onward have AC adapters on their power cords, so it will be next to impossible to fry your CPAP when you change to different voltages around the globe. If you don't know, though, call your provider or manufacturer—they will know instantly!

5) *Can I change my pressure? Will this stay the same forever?*

The reality is that the pressure on your machine has been prescribed to you by a sleep-medicine doctor. It's like being prescribed a drug. You can't just walk into a pharmacy and ask for hydromorphone when you have a prescription for codeine; the same goes for your prescribed pressure. If you are having problems getting used to your pressure, or if you feel as though you need it bumped up, you can simply call your sleep doctor and ask for a visit to discuss this. Unfortunately, your favourite RT can't just change it willy-nilly either, unless they have a standing order from your doctor that says they are allowed to change it. Will the pressure you start with be your forever pressure? Sometimes yes, sometimes no. As humans, we are constantly changing and adapting to new things. Some people end up needing pressure changes every now and then, and some people stay true to their original prescription pressure. Is one worse than the other? No, not at all. There is no "getting worse" or "getting better," the reality is that sometimes things change for no reason. And that's okay. You're okay. Everybody is okay.

6) *Do I have to use humidity?*

Using the humidifier part of your CPAP machine isn't mandatory. For some models, it needs to remain attached to the motor, but if you feel more comfortable not putting water in it and/or not turning on the heat at all, that is totally up to you. It's what we call a comfort setting, and the great thing about comfort settings is that you can choose whatever you like. Quite frankly, if there was a wrong answer to your comfort settings, you would not be allowed to change them! The majority of CPAP clients use the humidity on their machines, but that doesn't mean that *you* have to. Besides, you can save money by not buying the distilled water!

7) *What position should I sleep in? Can I still lie on my side?*

The answer is you can sleep in whatever position you want! There is such a large range of masks available to you, Goldilocks, that you will be able to find the one that is juuuust right. Most people with sleep apnea started sleeping on their side because their body learned that when they do this, the obstruction in their airway is less severe! It all comes down to gravity, so when we sleep on our back, the apnea is worse, and when we sleep on our side, it's a smidge better.

8) *All of this equipment is really expensive. How can I save some money?*

If you have health benefits from your employer or from the government, check there first. Most insurance companies will reimburse you for a mask, tube, water tub, and pack of filters every year. Sometimes, they will need a quote for approval before you can go ahead with the purchase. Your provider should provide this for you at no cost. Another great way to save some money is to purchase your equipment online. The benefit of buying in person is that you have access to experts who can help you buy the right items, which is why brick and mortar prices are higher than online prices. Also, buying masks

in person will usually allow you to take advantage of the

thirty-day mask exchange policy that stores will have with

the manufacturers. Online stores won't usually offer you

this, so you have to be certain what mask you need! If

you want help ordering supplies online, try getting in

touch with the vendor via telephone, and they can help

you out.

Chapter 9

The Grand Finale

Well that's the long and the short of it.

You, or your loved one who uses CPAP, are going to adapt and evolve. It's what we do, as humans. CPAP is meant to be a tool that enhances your life, not something that you need to be married to or fearful of. The symptoms of sleep apnea will start to disappear once regular CPAP use becomes a part of your life. Fewer headaches, less fatigue, less interrupted sleep, better memory, fewer rib injuries from your bed partner elbowing you at night, and less drowsiness can all be expected after starting CPAP.

We hope that this book has given you a bit of relief, especially if you were feeling any anxiety about starting CPAP. We know that a lot of people have a lot of questions, and sometimes there is just *so much* information, so having this book as a reference should give you peace of mind. You are not alone; there are communities out there and forums online where you can find other CPAP users who have just as many questions as you do!

Thank you for reading this book, we hope that we have reached our goal of CPAP MADE SIMPLE!

Kindest regards and happy sleeping!

RT4ME, your personal RTs!

NOTES:

84

My CPAP

My machine: ________________________________

Manufacturer: ________________________________

My pressure: ____

My mask: ________________________________

Size: ____________________________

My date of purchase: ____

My supplier:____

Copyright